PROTECT YOURSELF

Folic acid, a key member of the vitamin B complex, is often missing in the meat-centered processed food supply of Americans. Yet, within the last decade there has been a burgeoning of research emphasizing its curative and protective properties in a wide variety of conditions, including malignancies, cardiovascular disease, cervical dysplasia and severe birth defects.

This important booklet by a prominent doctor of nutritional medicine offers essential information about the role this valuable nutrient plays in a variety of disease states. Dr. Baker discusses food sources, supplement dosages, possible side effects and contraindications for folic acid and helps us to understand the unique role that folic acid plays in the body's biochemistry.

AF722931

ABOUT THE AUTHOR

Sidney MacDonald Baker, M.D. is a practicing physician in Weston, Connecticut. He graduated from Yale Medical School in 1964 and did specialty training in obstetrics and gynecology and pediatrics, in which he is board certified. He is also board certified in environmental medicine. He served in Chad, Africa, as a Peace Corps volunteer, has worked as a family practitioner in an H.M.O., was director of the Gesell Institute of Human Development, and for the last decade has been in private practice. He is co-author with Ilg and Ames of *Child Behavior* (Harper & Row, 1982) and *Your Ten to Fourteen Year Old* (Delacorte, 1988). He has published several popular and scientific articles about nutritional biochemistry.

FOLIC ACID

THE VITAL NUTRIENT THAT FIGHTS BIRTH DEFECTS CANCER AND HEART DISEASE

by Sidney M. Baker, M.D.

Keats Publishing, Inc. New Canaan, Connecticut

Folic Acid is not intended as medical advice. Its intent is solely informational and educational. Please consult a health professional should the need for one be indicated.

FOLIC ACID

ISBN: 0-87983-662-8

Printed in the United States of America

Good Health Guides are published by
Keats Publishing, Inc.
27 Pine Street (Box 876)
New Canaan, Connecticut 06840-0876

Contents

INTRODUCTION

Protection and tailoring. In the future, when we human beings finally learn to protect ourselves with nutritional supplements in the same way that we have learned to clothe ourselves with cloth and to shelter ourselves with houses, folic acid will be first on the list of top protective nutrients. In the future, when we human beings finally learn to tailor our nutrition to individual quirks as we have learned to fit our clothes and houses to our special needs, folic acid will be one of the nutrients for which many individuals have quirky needs.

The future is already here for some of us, but it will take another generation to achieve widespread acceptance of nutritional protection and tailoring. General recognition of the need for nutritional supplements is still limited, and folic acid's importance to health has not been widely publicized. Folic acid is much more important to our health than dozens of medications we hear advertised constantly. It does not, however, have a corporate sponsor. Moreover, the documentation supporting individual decisions to take folic acid is quite recent. Before the last decade most doctors were aware of only two important attributes of folic acid:

1. It is the only vitamin for which a moderately large dose requires a doctor's prescription—because high doses can mask vitamin B_{12} deficiency.
2. It is an important factor in the nutrition of bacteria, parasites and cancer cells. Certain antimicrobial and anticancer drugs work by interfering with the folic acid metabolism of the target germs or cancer cells.

The last decade has witnessed a burgeoning of research about the curative and protective properties of folic acid in a wide variety of conditions, including cardiovascular disease, malignancies and severe birth defects. The dosage of folic acid used for the treatment or prevention of these conditions has, in some instances, been far in excess of official dietary recommendations. Thus, "megavitamin therapy," which has been widely condemned in the official pronouncements of government and mainstream medicine, has in this instance gained acceptance. Even though very large doses of vitamins may be used for the treatment of certain rare diseases of metabolism, we are most often urged to fulfill our nutritional requirements through a "balanced diet."

For the first time the official recommendations for folic acid could not be realistically reached with dietary modification alone.

A word about diet. When I was five years old I went to a birthday party where my playmate's mother served us liver, onions and peas. It was during World War II when discarding food was unpatriotic. My mother also let me know that not finishing what was on my plate was inconsiderate of those nonwarring peoples who were starving. When I was to be a guest at someone else's house, these rules would achieve maximum force. I had never been offered liver before, and, after dutifully choking it down at the party, I took an oath over my empty plate that I would never eat liver again. I have remained faithful to my oath. Some tabulations of the folic acid content of the average composite American diet include small amounts of liver eaten by the "average" person. Liver accounts for the lion's share of the daily folic acid calculation when it is included as part of the imaginary "average" diet. The disproportionate contribution of liver to the averages convinces me that I could not consume substantial amounts of folic acid without supplements, even though I do like spinach which is a rich source of folic acid.

You may get the impression from this booklet that I, like many physicians, am a pill pusher, indifferent to the value of a good diet. I am not. The first steps in health are good breathing and good eating. By good eating, I mean the consumption of tasty, varied, fresh, lean, nutrient-dense, unprocessed, unrefined and unadulterated foods. The point is, however, that evidence is mounting that at least some of us need to go beyond dietary excellence and to supplement with certain minerals, fatty acids, amino acids, vitamins and accessory nutritional factors that do not fall neatly into any of the above categories.

Sides. When meeting a stranger who asks what kind of doctor I am, I still grope for an explanation. I know my questioner is looking for a specialty, but I characterize myself more by my point of view than by a specialty. My first realization that I had a point of view came at 2 A.M. one Sunday morning when, as a senior medical student, I was serving as a subintern in pediatrics. That night, my job was to get permission for a routine autopsy from the parents of a 2 year old who had just died of meningitis. The hospital's accreditation depended on having a certain percentage of autopsies, and so pressure was placed on the medical staff to get permission for one whenever possible. Getting permission served the goals of the medical hierarchy of which I was at the bottom. In this particular instance, an autopsy was unlikely to reveal anything new about my patient's devastating and well-defined illness. So, as soon as I glimpsed their opposition, I sided with the family and did not press them for permission.

From then on, I knew that I would encounter many situations when there would be two sides with an element of conflict. Sometimes I have found that the conflict is between points of view that embrace change more or less easily. At other times the discord is between private versus public motives. For example, children are immunized against German measles in order to lessen the public exposure of pregnant women to the virus. I encourage immunization of children to limit the spread of the virus to pregnant women, but for a given child I might opt against immunization when it offers no direct advantage to him or her, especially if everyone else is doing it.

With regard to folic acid, public policy at present is to recommend folic acid consumption in the range of the RDA (Recommended Daily Allowance) of less than 200 micrograms daily. A private decision to take more would not have the same antisocial flavor as refusing a German measles immunization, but a conservative medical professional may still view it as an unwise exercise of individual discretion. The patient's side often has to do with a looser, more speculative and speedier interpretation of the available information as reflected in the following patient's question: "If folic acid has been shown to be effective in protecting against colon cancer, bronchial cancer, esophageal cancer and malignant changes in the cervix of the uterus, wouldn't it be reasonable to take supplements of folic acid as a precaution against these or other forms of cancer that worry me because of my family and occupational history?"

Balance. Most of what I have learned in 30 years of doctoring has come from listening to my patients and trying to find the answers to two simple questions that are raised by what a patient tells me. The first question is: "Could this person have some special need, which, if met, would clear up or improve the situation?" The second question is: "Could this person have too much of something that does not agree with him or her (a toxin, allergen or germ), which if reduced or eliminated would clear up or improve the situation?" These questions are different from "What is the diagnosis?" The two questions have to do with balance—enough of the good things and not too much of the bad things—and are useful questions no matter what name (diagnosis) one puts on the person's problems.

So it was with Senior Pilot Mack Winger when he came to ask my opinion after he totaled his Mercedes on a bridge abutment. The problem was that he kept falling asleep at the wrong moment. "Narcolepsy," said the neurologist whom Captain Winger had consulted. Indeed, the story fit the textbook definition of this extreme form of inopportune somnolence. But Captain Winger did not want to take the medication prescribed. He just did not like the way he felt on "speed," which is how he referred to the various brands of stimulant medication prescribed by the neurologist. I began my workup of Captain Winger by checking his blood vitamin levels at the laboratory of Herman Baker (no relation), who is the foremost expert in blood vitamin determination. The folic acid level was 3.2, with the normal range being between 5 and 24. Taking folic acid supplements of 2 to 3 milligrams* (mg) per day alleviated Captain Winger's problem by about 70 percent. Other kinds of intervention helped improve the problem further so that he was able to function safely no matter what kind of craft he was steering.

Treating the individual versus treating the diagnosis. There are two reasons for sketching Captain Winger's story. One is to illustrate the point about balance: making sure that no matter what chronic problem a person has, that I consider whether he or she is missing something for which there is a special need. The other reason is to illustrate a point about diagnosis. In many instances, the characteristics of the person with the diagnosis are just as important in getting to a proper treatment as are the characteristics of the diagnosed disease. It would be wrong to see Captain Winger's case as the cure of narcolepsy with folic acid. There are lots of people with narcolepsy who do not have folic acid deficiency and whose narcolepsy would not benefit from folic acid supplementation. And Captain Winger still had a tendency toward somnolence after his folic acid deficiency was treated. But his tendency was so minimized that it was manageable without drugs. Folic acid was a treatment for Captain Winger as an individual, and it was not a treatment aimed at his diagnosis of narcolepsy.

Books have chapters, bodies don't. As you read in this booklet about various particular problems, remember that this arrangement has to do with the way research is conducted and books are written. It makes it seem as if the human body is made out of chapters like a medical textbook. But it is not. It is a unity that we try to understand by considering its different parts. If you read on, you will learn that folic acid's role in chemistry is so fundamental that it would be silly to think that it is important in only certain parts or conditions of the body. The parts and conditions of the body that have recently burst into the medical literature in relation to folic acid are the tip of an iceberg that will

*There are 1000 milligrams (mg) in a gram. A drop of water weighs about 50 milligrams. There are 1000 micrograms (mcg) in a milligram. The dose of folic acid that is usually found in over-the-counter vitamins is 400 mcg, which is the same as 0.4 mg. The maximum dose that can be sold without a prescription is 0.8 mg or 800 mcg.

become revealed over the next generation. Enough ice is showing now in the late 1990s for a prudent person to make personal decisions about folic acid supplementation.

Deficiency? Finally, you may be a little confused about whether I am talking about folic acid deficiency or taking folic acid in therapeutic amounts above and beyond that needed to correct a deficiency. If a woman needs to take 15 mg of folic acid daily to cure a chronically persistent, severely abnormal Pap smear (cervical dysplasia), is it because she had a "deficiency" in the same sense as 0.4 mg corrects all tests that are used to diagnose folic acid deficiency? I doubt that Mother Nature draws a clear line, so you and I will remain confused about the strict definition of deficiency in regard to folic acid. The notion that vitamins are needed only to correct measurable vitamin deficiencies has, however, been a firm medical dogma for the past three generations. Within that dogma, deficiency has meant a low blood level or equivalent measure of folic acid function. The doses that I advocate to control or prevent the conditions that follow are designed to correct a need that is not currently called a "deficiency."

MALIGNANCIES

A hot potato. In 1993 I gave a prescription for 5 mg of folic acid to a patient who had consulted me concerning ways to combat a cancer of his voice box that had spread to the local lymph nodes. Folic acid pills do not yet come in a 5 mg size unless a pharmacist makes them up specially. I apparently did not explain carefully enough to my patient that he should fill his prescription at a particular pharmacy that made up 5 mg folic acid capsules for my patients. He took my prescription to his local pharmacist who looked at it and asked with a certain edge: "What kind of doctor is this?" "A licensed one," replied my patient, who is a man of considerable warmth, dignity and independent spirit. A short discussion ensued in which my patient invited the pharmacist to phone me. Instead, the pharmacist declared, "In all my years of pharmacy I have never seen such a thing," and, pronouncing it "out of bounds," thrust the prescription back across the counter at my patient.

Pharmacists, whose patience and thoroughness often compensate for my haste and illegibility, are the last professionals from whom I would expect such arrogant bluster. But vitamins do get people's dander up. And so, of course, for better reasons, does cancer. When mentioned together—vitamins and cancer—during the last few decades, most physicians would be so deafened by quacking noises that they could not consider the subject carefully. You should be prepared for an understandable negative reaction if you ask your physician for a prescription for folic acid in an effort to reduce cancer risks. Most of us were told years ago by our professors that vitamins are a bunch of nonsense. Authoritative editorials have proclaimed the taking of vitamins beyond what you can get from a "healthy diet" to be medically unsound and have reinforced the disdain of many physicians for vitamin supplementation. The situation has only begun to change. A harried doctor does know that at least one anticancer drug, methotrexate, works by antagonizing folic acid functions in cancer cells. He or she may have gone on to suppose that if one way to kill cancer cells is to deprive them of folic acid, then maybe folic acid would encourage cancer. The paradox is so confusing, the thought of promoting cancer is so scary, and sins of commission (giving folic acid) are so much more worrisome than sins of omission that many physicians hesitate to prescribe folic acid when cancer is present.

Epithelium, megaloblastosis and dysplasia. Epithelium is a medical term for the cells that cover the inner and outer surfaces of the body, such as the skin, the lining of the lung's branching tubules, the digestive tract and the urinary and reproductive passages (*epi* = outer, *thelium* = covering).

Other tissues of the body, such as parts of the nervous system, are linked because they were derived from the same parts of the early embryo as the epithelium. The kinds of cancers whose prevention or correction in early stages has been most clearly associated with folic acid supplementation are the cancers of epithelial cells. When cells change in a cancerous direction, they take on an appearance under the microscope in which certain parts become enlarged and misshapen. When applied to cancer cells, this change is called dysplasia (*dys* = abnormal, *plasia* = growth). A similar appearance called megaloblastosis (*megalo* = large, *blast* = a cellular growth stage, *osis* = process) occurs in cells in the blood and epithelium in the presence of folic acid and/or vitamin B_{12} deficiency. As early as 1954, the cancer susceptibility of individuals with pernicious anemia (from folic acid and/or B_{12} deficiency) was discussed in terms of the relationship between megaloblastosis and dysplasia.[1] The relationship is now known to be a close one in that both are responsive to folic acid supplementation with a lowering of cancer risk.

Surfaces. Epithelium has to do with surfaces. So how much surface do you have? If you were to make a body suit to cover every inch of your skin, you would need between 1 and 2 square yards of material to cover everything for an average or large adult. That takes care of your outside epithelium. What about the inner surfaces (on which you exchange materials such as air, food and water with the outside world)? Pull down your lower lip and estimate its inner surface area based on dimensions of about 1 by 2 inches: 2 square inches. If you continue this measuring as you come to your tongue, you may observe that your tongue is not smooth, but is covered by little bumpy projections. If you are serious about measuring the true surface, you will have to measure down and in between and up around all the little bumps and projections. Upon reaching the stomach, especially the small intestine, you will discover (with the aid of a microscope) that the bumpiness gets very complicated, so that tiny fingerlike projections are themselves the bearers of teensy weensy fingerlike projections. The total surface area of the gut as measured by including the surface of all the bumps and projections comes out to be about the size of a tennis court. All epithelium. The same can be said for your lung's inner surface. But here the architecture has to do with branching tubules instead of bumpy projections. Knowing that these epithelial surface areas are both very large and very subject to wear and tear, it is less surprising that they are susceptible to cancerous changes that can be modified or cured with a substance (folic acid) that is intimately connected with healthy cell growth.

Abnormal Pap Smears

Prevention and treatment. The cervix (from the Latin word for neck) is the part of a woman's uterus that extends half an inch or so into the upper part of the vagina. An opening, which appears like a constricted cleft in the center of a 1-inch sized smooth pink donut, becomes the passageway that opens when a baby is delivered from the womb. In a nonpregnant mature woman, the canal of the cervix allows for the exit of menstrual blood and the entry of sperm. The surface of the cervix surrounding the hole can be gently scraped with a narrow instrument, such as a disposable wooden or plastic paddle, and if the instrument is promptly rubbed on a glass microscope slide, cells from the cervix can be examined. Normally, these cells have the appearance of transparent chips or flakes or scales, each with a small compact granule (the nucleus) within it. The cells are from the epithelium of the cervix.

A method for collecting, preparing, staining and examining the cells of the cervix was developed by Dr. Papanicolau and is known as a Pap smear. Cervical cells examined by this method reveal changes that reflect inflammation of the cervix and various stages on the way to cancer. One of the changes that occurs when cells go through the stages leading to cancer is in the size of the nucleus. The enlargement of the cell and of its nucleus is similar to megaloblastic changes that are seen in cells when there is a deficiency of folic acid or vitamin B_{12}. Typically, such changes have been associated with the blood cells—hence the term *megaloblastic anemia* to describe enlargement of blood cells accompanied by a net drop in the number of red blood cells in people with folic acid or vitamin B_{12} deficiency.

In 1973 N. Whitehead[2] reported observing that abnormalities in cervical cells seen in Pap smears of women taking birth control pills were cured when the women took supplements of folic acid. The similarity of these megaloblastic changes to dysplasia that may be the precursor of cancerous changes led to further speculation that folic acid deficiency might play a role in cancer of the cervix. In 1982 Dr. Charles E. Butterworth, Jr., of the University of Alabama carried out a trial of folic acid treatment in women with abnormal Pap smears. The results of the trial in 47 women suggested an association between cervical dysplasia and folic acid deficiency. Dr. Butterworth wondered at the time whether the megaloblastic changes of folic acid deficiency might be confused with the appearance of a precancerous condition. Now it is quite clear that the megaloblastic changes are indeed precancerous.

Based on Butterworth's original report,[3] during the last ten years I have given large doses of folic acid (10 to 20 mg daily) to women in whom a persistently abnormal Pap smear was either the main reason for their consulting me or was something that came up in their history, I have not seen a single treatment failure. My patients have included dozens of women, some with multiple abnormal Pap smears and biopsies over periods of months or years. None of the women I have observed were taking birth control pills during the time of folic acid treatment. About half the cases of abnormal Pap smears will return to normal without any specific treatment, so it may be that my experience represents a statistical fluke. Nevertheless, I have found that the use of 10 to 20 mg of folic acid is a sure bet, and since it usually works within a month or two, I believe it should be the first step in women with abnormal Pap smears.

For example, a few years ago my daughter told me that one of her best friends at college was terrified because she had had a series of abnormal Pap smears and cervical biopsies and conizations (in which a cone of tissue is surgically removed from the circumference of the cervix), with no improvement in the premalignant condition that was revealed with each procedure. Her gynecologist had started talking about removing her uterus, a devastating prospect for a 21-year-old woman. After examining her and her previous records, I suggested that she take 15 to 20 mg of folic acid daily in addition to a multivitamin for a month before her next gynecological examination. At that examination, no abnormal cells could be found in her cervix.

My own experience may be a statistical fluke because Dr. Butterworth and his group carried out a study[4] in which 235 women with abnormal Pap smears were treated for six months with either folic acid or a placebo (10 mg of vitamin C). Of 199 women completing the study, about 60 percent of women in both groups had normal Pap smears at the end of the six-month period. Eighty percent of the women in the study were taking birth control pills both before and during the study. There was no significant difference in the placebo-treated versus the folic acid-treated groups with respect to measurement of red blood cell (RBC) folic acid levels or the results of treatment. Women with evidence of infection with a common genital viral infection (human papilloma virus or HPV) had lower levels of RBC folic acid at the beginning of the study than women with HPV infection. At the end of the study, there was only a mild suggestion in the statistics that the folic acid treatment reduced the incidence of HPV infection.

The results of the study are puzzling in light of other studies in which folic acid is clearly correlated with risk of cervical cancer. Dr. Butterworth's group did the treatment study because a previous case-control study[5] had shown a significant correlation between low RBC folic acid levels and risk factors for cervical dysplasia, especially HPV infection. Dr. Butterworth reached the conclusion that low red blood cell folic acid levels enhance the effect of other risk factors (number of sex partners, number of pregnancies, oral contraceptive use, and HPV infection and cigarette smoking) for cervical cancer. Women with low folic acid levels were five times more likely to have cervical dysplasia than those who did not have low folic acid levels. The protective effect of high folic acid levels makes it easier for women to decide what to do about supplementation, even though there is a lack of reliable published information in support of taking folic acid supplements to treat abnormal Pap smears. At the moment, there is no reliable way for a given woman to determine her need for folic acid supplementation for prevention of cervical dysplasia. A low red blood cell folic acid level would be a helpful indicator that a woman is in a higher risk group, but it would not be completely decisive in the question of whether or not to take supplements.

Cervical cancer is the ninth most common cause of cancer deaths among women in the United States and is six times more frequent in parts of South America.[6] The economic and human costs of detection and surgical treatment of precancerous cervical lesions are enormous, and the incidence of death, despite widespread efforts at early detection and treatment, is tragic. If supplementation with folic acid were effective in preventing some or all of this disease, the taking of supplements by all women would be a bargain. Before public health authorities recommend this approach, more research data are needed as well as an ideological shift. The prevailing idea about supplements is that they are needed only to prevent deficiency diseases. Cervical dysplasia has not been thought of as a deficiency disease. The idea that supplements of a vitamin or combinations of vitamins offer protection against various diseases has not yet become part of the accepted way of thinking among public health policymakers.

In the meantime, what about private health authorities, namely, you? While waiting for more information to appear, is it prudent to take folic acid supplements in doses of 5 to 15 mg, which is well above the recommended daily allowance of less than 0.2 mg daily? Most medical authorities today would opt to wait for much more information before recommending high-dose folic acid supplementation to a given person.

When face to face with a patient in my office, I have no trouble recommending that she supplement with folic acid for preventive purposes, and I continue to treat abnormal Pap smears with high doses of folic acid. My job in writing this booklet is to acquaint you with the facts and to indicate where you can get more information, not to make any specific recommendation about what you should do. If you take birth control pills, there is good evidence supporting supplementation with folic acid and vitamin B_6.[7] As I implied previously in discussing Dr. Butterworth's studies, birth control pills increase your needs for both vitamins, and lacking supplementation leaves you at greater risk for developing cervical dysplasia while taking birth control pills. If you have an infection with HPV, the idea of taking large doses of folic acid seems to make pretty good sense.

Colon Cancer

Antidote to a drug or protection from disease? In 1989 B. A. Lashner[8] reported a case-controlled study showing that folic acid supplementation (1 mg per day) reduced colon cancer by 62 percent in patients with ulcerative colitis as compared with those patients who were not given folic acid supplementation. The drug *sulfasalazine,* which all the patients were taking, was implicated as a factor because it interferes with folic acid absorption. Lashner's recommendation was clear cut: folic acid supplementation during sulfasalazine administration to prevent cancer in patients with ulcerative colitis. If this study were the only one pointing to a relationship between a relative lack of folic acid and epithelial dysplasia, it would be easier to keep Dr. Lashner's recommendation limited to cases of ulcerative colitis treated with sulfasalazine. Given that there is broad evidence that supplementation with folic acid reduces risks for epithelial cancers, it would be difficult for me not to recommend folic acid supplementation to a patient with chronic inflammation of the bowel, while at the same time undertaking an investigation to find out what is causing the inflammation.

Lung and Esophageal Cancer

In 1988 D. Heimberger, an associate of Dr. Butterworth in the Departments of Nutrition Sciences and Medicine at the

University of Alabama, reported a double-blind study in which either a placebo or daily doses of 10 mg of folic acid and 0.5 mg of vitamin B_{12} (as hydroxycobalamin) were given to tobacco smokers with precancerous changes in their bronchial tissues. The authors were unable to conclude which of the two vitamins used might account for the significant improvement seen in the precancerous changes of the vitamin-treated group as compared with the placebo-treated group.

Part of the logic behind the study has to do with the observation that chromosomal breaks are frequently observed in cancer cells and are associated with a failure in proper methylation of the DNA molecules of chromosomes. Since methylation is a function of folic acid and since vitamin B_{12} is folic acid's partner in this activity, it was reasonable to use both nutrients together in the study. In fact, on both clinical and biochemical grounds, it seems awkward to give just one of these two nutrients in nutritional studies because they are so interdependent at one of B_{12}'s "workstations" in human biochemistry.

A scientific principle guides researchers and clinicians when they are trying to figure out how things work. This guiding doctrine, the so-called Principle of Parsimony, insists on a careful effort to identify the fewest, preferably single, causal factors in any given outcome.

Take the case of scurvy, the disease caused by vitamin C deficiency. In 1546 the explorer Jacques Cartier was wintering over on the St. Lawrence River near the present-day city of Quebec. His ship was frozen into the river ice, and the ship's crew was subsisting on ship's stores of grains and hard tack. As winter progressed, scurvy began to take its toll despite various efforts at prayer and the medicinal remedies of the time. Loosened teeth, reopened old wounds, skin sores, mental aberrations and fatigue led to death for several crew members before a friendly Native American heard about the troubles. He let Cartier know that there was a simple remedy for the problem, which was well known to Native American medicine. He showed Cartier's men how to make an infusion from the boughs of the northern white cedar tree. After drinking the infusion, the few afflicted men who dared to try the novel treatment were restored to health within days. The others waited for a double-blind placebo controlled study to be published in a peer reviewed medical journal before attempting the cure.

Just kidding! The truth is that the lives of Cartier's men were saved by the simple remedy with its generous concentration of vitamin C. A specimen of the northern white cedar was taken back to France on Cartier's homeward voyage. It was the first tree ever imported to Europe from North America. The King of France named it *arbor vitae* (the tree of life) to celebrate its rescue of Cartier's expedition. In the case of the treatment taken by Cartier's men, vitamin C and only vitamin C was clearly the key element in curing scurvy.

A parsimonious approach favors economy and logic. The rule is particularly appropriate to the use of medications or other treatments for acute illness in which a single cause can be identified. In the case of drug treatments, it makes sense to give only one at a time in order to achieve a desired effect so that, at the very least, an adverse reaction can be attributed to the drug without delay. When it comes to research or treatment of patients, giving two or more drugs at once is usually frowned upon because it may lead to confusion about which drug is working, and it risks overtreatment.

When I first incorporated some knowledge of my patients' biochemical needs and quirks into my practice, I felt uneasy about giving several nutrients at once because I was haunted by the Principle of Parsimony which had been such an important dogma of my training. Biochemistry, however, is all interconnected. One simply cannot conceive of using nutrients as if they were drugs, even though minerals, vitamins, amino acids and fatty acids may sometimes have effects that are practically druglike. The interdependence of nutrients makes it sensible to prescribe pairs or groups of nutrients that are known to have cooperative biochemical effects. Such an approach may make good biochemical sense, as well as being nontoxic (which is not always true of combining several drugs), but it does not fit well into the models established for acceptable research, in which only a single variable is the preferred target of investigation.

In other words, Dr. Heimberger and his colleagues were

rather daring to undertake an experiment in which two nutrients were used together. It appears that a combination of courage and plain biochemical sense guided them, and we are all the beneficiaries of their example, which may take hold in further nutritional studies. You may be aware of the recent publication of the failure of vitamins C and/or E to influence the outcome of disease in a group of Finnish smokers. It was argued that antioxidants should have a protective effect in smokers. Vitamins C and E, however, are only two members of a whole group of nutrients which work together to provide antioxidant defense. Antioxidants are like a ladder, in which each rung is a necessary element in the success of the device. Would it make sense to take one or two rungs out of a ladder, show that they, alone or in a pair, are of no help in climbing to the roof and conclude that ladders are useless?

Local tissue difference in folic acid needs. Low folic acid levels appear to be associated with cancer of the esophagus. A very high incidence of esophageal cancer has been observed in parts of South Africa. Factors thought to contribute to the high incidence are the use of tobacco, alcohol, grain contaminated with a particular fungus and a seasonal lack of fresh produce, combined with a general state of poverty. Studies of cells taken from the esophagus of individuals in this population have shown a cellular appearance consistent with folic acid deficiency.[9] The authors propose that some local tissues (that is, in the surface tissues of the esophagus) are deficient in folic acid. The local tissue deficiencies are not always reflected by other measures of folic acid in the blood or other tissues. The idea of local tissue deficiency of folic acid has also been presented by Heimberger,[10] who reviews the evidence that folic acid deficiency should predispose tissues to cancerous transformation because

1. Folic acid performs a critical function making and repairing chromosomes.
2. Chromosomal damage of the kind associated with cancer occurs in cells that are grown in cultures when the culture medium contains low levels of folic acid.
3. Smokers with low blood levels of folic acid have more

chromosomes with greater susceptibility to damage than smokers or nonsmokers with normal folic acid levels.

4. Cancer occurs more frequently among people with low folic acid intake in their diet.
5. There is a higher risk of cancer in people who have taken methotrexate, a cancer drug that works by creating a folic acid deficiency, so that patients treated successfully with methotrexate may be at higher risk for developing a subsequent cancer.

Heimberger points out that it is difficult to explain the development of localized cancerous changes without considering that the local tissues may have a special need for more folic acid than neighboring or distant parts of the body.

If there are local tissue differences in folic acid needs, then blood tests are less decisive in folic acid assessment in any given human being. Add the fact that all human beings are different in their overall needs for folic acid and you arrive at a situation that is confusing for both the physician advising the patient and the patient trying to sort out the possible advantages of supplementation. The situation is even more confusing for those charged with making policy that is meant to affect everyone in a population uniformly.

Cancer Summary

Cancer is usually the result of the interaction of various risk factors, including genetic predisposition, viral infections, exposure to environmental toxins and nutritional and other aspects of each person's life experience. It would be simple-minded to think of folic acid deficiency as "the cause" of anyone's cancer. On the other hand, it would be wise to heed the accumulated evidence suggesting that folic acid needs affect the ways cancer risk factors are expressed. Suppose that one person has a relatively high cancer risk because of an inherited tendency or because of exposures to chemicals that predispose to cancer. Would such a person lower his or her risks of cancer by taking extra amounts of folic acid? Suppose, on the other hand, that a person has no inherited cancer risks and no environmental exposures, but eats a diet that is deficient in folic acid. Would such a person be at risk for cancer because of folic acid deficiency, or would he or she simply experience fatigue or other relatively benign symptoms of folic acid deficiency? Both questions are unanswerable at present.

It is unlikely that the kinds of cancer involved in the folic acid story are limited to the ones I have mentioned, although epithelial cancers will probably remain the cancers with the strongest correlation to folic acid quirks and deficiencies. Whatever kinds of cancer eventually join the list will likely tend to be cancers of the body's busiest tissues: that is, those subject to wear and tear and the need for constant and rapid cellular replacement. Most physicians will probably wait for those who make public policy to recommend folic acid supplementation as a cancer preventative; such a recommendation may await better tests to identify those individuals who are at risk for folic acid deficiency cancer.

We physicians want, at the very least, to do no harm to our patients. Such an impulse often weighs the scales in favor of withholding any treatment when there is the slightest question of safety. The question regarding safety sometimes arises from our unfamiliarity with a subject, and nutrition is a subject about which physicians are often poorly informed. We are trained to withhold treatment when none is indicated; that inclination is strengthened by an awareness that doing nothing may *seem* safer than doing something.

I recommend high doses of folic acid to any patient who expresses concern about cancer. Depending on how it fits in with other biochemical priorities that may arise, at some point I will raise the question of cancer risk factors with my patients. I personally have a family history of cancer myself; therefore I take 5 mg of folic acid daily.

PREGNANCY AND FETAL DEFECTS

The odds. Out of every hundred babies born, about three have some kind of imperfection detectable as they begin life. One of the three has a defect that results in a major disappointment or at least a challenge to the parents, other family members and, of course, the afflicted person. Many birth defects can be treated so that their effects do not become a permanent handicap. Others, however, are very difficult to repair. Many birth defects can be understood in terms of abnormalities in the baby's chromosomes, or injuries to the embryo after pregnancy has begun. Injuries resulting from virus infections, exposures to drugs, hormones, toxins, radiation and other stresses are expressed to different degrees and in different ways depending on the timing of the exposure. One particular group of injuries to the developing embryo results from the failure of the neural tube to close.

A stuck zipper. During its first few weeks of development, a human embryo becomes a tiny disk with a groove. The groove then becomes a tube as the groove is closed from end to end as if the edges were joined by a zipper. This process occurs in the tissue that is to become the digestive tract on the front side of the embryo and separately on the back in the tissue that is to become the brain, spinal cord and their coverings. Failure of closure of the brain and spinal cord tube, called the neural tube, results in several birth defects called neural tube defects.

The defect may be minor and result in only a small, insignificant gap in one layer of the coverings of the upper or, usually, lower spinal cord. Often, however, the defect is major and results in a devastating injury. The severe injuries range in expression from a more or less complete absence of the brain (anencephaly) to a wide opening at the base of the spine of the newborn (meningomyelocoele). Babies with anencephaly may survive for days to months, depending on the intensity of the care provided. Those with meningomyelocoele are at risk for infections of the spinal fluid, which may be exposed to the air if a delicate sac covering the spinal nerves is ruptured at birth or in the newborn period before it can be repaired by plastic surgery. Even if the meningomyelocoele is repaired, the nerves leaving the base of the spinal cord remain without function and the afflicted person experiences paralysis of the legs and lack of control over bowels and bladder. Other names for this condition or variations in its location are *spina bifida* and *encephalocoele.*

The incidence of this defect was observed to be high in certain geographic areas, such as Wales and Ireland, where people were genetically no different from Welsh and Irish people living elsewhere, such as North America or Australia where the incidence of this birth defect was not so high. An environmental cause was suspected.

In 1976 Drs. Smithells, Sheppard and Schorah of the Department of Medicine at the University of Leeds in England reported their study[11] of serum folic acid, red cell folic acid, white blood cell vitamin C, riboflavin saturation index and serum vitamin A during the first three months of pregnancy in over 900 women of whom six gave birth to babies with neural tube defects. Both measures of folic acid and the white blood cell levels of vitamin C were lower in these six women than in the women who did not give birth to babies with neural tube defects. Despite the small numbers, the differences in folic acid levels were so marked that they could only have occurred by chance within less than once in a thousand times. The differences in vitamin C levels could have occurred by chance less than five times out of a hundred, which is the conventionally accepted point where one can reject the notion that chance explains an observed pattern of events.

After publication of the findings of the University of Leeds group, only a very few physicians accepted the fact that the folic acid measures almost certainly defined a difference between the women who gave birth to babies with neural tube defects and those who did not. Not many physicians began to urge women of childbearing age to ensure a generous intake of folic acid while further research continued. The implications of the initial report were important from the standpoint of public policy, which, at the time, never promoted the widespread use of any vitamin supplement. The medical profession, which tends to be skeptical of any claim that nutritional supplements can alter diseases, generally took the position that more research was needed to prove the connection between folic acid needs and neural tube defects.

Now, nearly two decades after the initial reports, public policy, as reflected in the recommendations of governmental bodies and authorities in obstetrics in the United Kingdom, the United States and most other developed countries, has endorsed folic acid supplementation for women entering pregnancy as a means of preventing neural tube defects.

The most decisive study on the question was carried out by the Medical Research Vitamin Study Research Group in the United Kingdom.[12] It was conducted at 33 centers in 7 countries to explore neural tube defect prevention by giving women various treatments around the time of conception. One group was supplemented with folic acid alone, another with a mixture of seven other vitamins (A, C, D, B_1, B_2, B_3 as niacinamide and B_6), a third was given both folic acid and the seven other vitamins, and a fourth group received a placebo that contained neither folic acid nor the other supplements. Over 1800 women who were at risk of a pregnancy with a neural tube defect participated in the study. Each woman was assigned to one of the treatment groups at random. Neither she nor those providing the supplements knew which regimen she was given. The results of the study showed a 72 percent protective effect of the folic acid supplementation without any protective effect from the other vitamins. There was no demonstrable harm observed from the folic acid supplementation, which was given at a dosage of 4.0 mg daily.

The conclusion of the study was that it could "now be firmly recommended" that women who have had a baby with neural tube defect should take folic acid supplementation to prevent another and that women of childbearing age should consume a diet containing an adequate amount of folic acid.

Does it strike you that the recommendation of the Medical Research Vitamin Study Research Group is quite timid? It exemplifies the difference between public policy and the choices available to a given individual. The Research Group is constrained by scientific caution to limit its recommendations to the bare minimum that are supported by the specific outcomes of the research. You, as a woman who might become pregnant, might, however, make a private decision to take a folic acid supplement, even though you have not yet had a baby with a neural tube defect. The demonstrated safety of doses in the neighborhood of 4.0 mg and the effectiveness of doses of 0.8 mg[13] might lead to a personal decision to take supplements in the rage of 0.8 to 4.0 mg daily to be on the safe side. The weight of evidence seen in the light of the very high stakes of having a baby with a life-threatening and permanent disability might lead you to make your choice about folic acid supplementation quite promptly.

Your physician might be more or less knowledgeable about the details of the various studies of folic acid and neural tube defects, and he or she might simply be familiar with the recommendations of the medical and public health policymakers. In the United States the U.S. Public Health Service recommends supplementation of 0.4 mg of folic acid beginning at least at the time of conception. It took the Public Health Service a year to come up with its recommendation following the issue of guidelines by the United States Center for Disease Control and Prevention, which stated its policy within weeks of the publication of the report of the Medical Research Vitamin Study Research Group. The slow pace and timidity of committees that recommend public policy is understandable considering that their decisions often have to do with drugs, which have a different level of risk than do nutrients.

The slow pace and caution of official recommendations in therapeutic nutrition should alert you as a consumer and me as a physician that we may be shortchanging ourselves if we simply wait for "them" to decide what is the best nutritional policy for each of us. There is presently a rapid growth of information concerning the potential of nutritional factors to mitigate illness. There is also a kind of rearguard action on the part of numerous experts who have decried nutrition as medical quackery for years and have a strong stake in that position.

CARDIOVASCULAR DISEASE

Warnings: If you have early-onset cardiovascular disease, your blood should be checked for your homocysteine level. If it is elevated, folic acid supplementation is very likely to bring it down along with your risk for heart attack, stroke and other blood vessel problems. Homocysteine (it rhymes with pristine) is an amino acid that is a central player in the body's methylation (single-carbon) chemistry. Homocysteine builds up in some individuals who have an inborn error of metabolism; yet the defect is rarely expressed in such an extreme degree that it results in the severe incapacitating disease called *homocysteinuria.* People with homocysteinuria have, among a variety of problems, early onset of cardiovascular disease in which blood vessels become blocked, causing heart attack, stroke and other problems that occur when an important organ is deprived of its blood supply.

Is there a spectrum? Considering that defects in single-carbon chemistry were found to have such a severe impact on cardiovascular health, the question came up as to whether there might be a spectrum of homocysteine problems outside of what we define as the disease. It turns out to be so, and individuals with mild homocysteine problems are susceptible to early-onset vascular problems. A group of researchers from the University of Lund Hospital in Sweden[14] evaluated 72 individuals who came to the hospital with occlusion of the arteries that supply blood to the brain and or legs. Their study was based on an understanding of the connection between vascular disease and homocysteine problems which has existed for the past two decades and which is fully accepted in the scientific community. Sixty-four percent of the group had abnormal homocysteine metabolism, in most instances because they carried the trait for homocysteinuria. (A man and a woman who each carry a trait may have children with the full-blown disease.)

Playing the odds. In making the diagnosis of abnormal homocysteine metabolism, the researchers found that the homocysteine problem was revealed in more than half of their patients only when methionine loading was done before measurement of homocysteine levels. Methionine is an essential amino acid which is transformed into homocysteine in two chemical steps. Homocysteine is subsequently used as a raw material for making other important molecules. It is also recycled back to form methionine by a different path than the one from which it came. Vitamin B_6, vitamin B_{12} and folic acid are all partners in the recycling of the homocysteine to methionine, in which a single-carbon unit (methyl group) is picked up by the homocysteine.

By giving vitamin B_6 and folic acid to their patients, the researchers were able to normalize the homocysteine levels. They concluded that a substantial share of patients with early-onset vascular disease have a problem with homocysteine metabolism that contributes to the disease. They point out that the problem can be corrected or improved easily and without side effects.

How early is early? By their definition, "early onset" means before age 55. Vascular problems are very common in industrialized countries. The causes have to do with diet and other environmental factors as well as genetics. Whereas the cost of vascular disease to our society is enormous, the cost of checking for homocysteine problems is small. A blood test for homocysteine runs about $100 in most laboratories. So far there has not been a public health recommendation that we all get checked for homocysteine with methionine loading. I think, however, that it is prudent for one to get checked for homocysteine at least once. The other option is simply to take generous amounts of folic acid and some form of vitamin B_6 just in case. If you are thinking about covering your bets this way, what you really want to know is whether the homocysteine problem is rare or common. The authors of a recent study[15] on the effects of vitamin B_6 in reducing the incidence of heart attacks based their finding on the ability of vitamin B_6 to lower homocysteine levels. Other studies[16] support the idea that most individuals can lower homocysteine levels by enriching their diet with foods or supplements that provide folic acid in doses of 5 mg daily, vitamin B_6 in doses of 50 mg daily and vitamin B_{12} in doses that depend a good deal on how well one absorbs oral supplementation. B_{12} supplementation can vary from 100 mcg daily by mouth to 1000 mcg by injection every two to four weeks.

The first observations concerning the relationship between homocysteinuria and cardiovascular disease go back to the 1960s.[17] At that time, researchers began to recognize a growing number of rare inborn metabolic diseases that could be modified or treated with large doses of certain vitamins. The vitamins worked not because "vitamins are good for you," but because they function as facilitators (co-enzymes) of certain steps in biochemical reactions. When there is a faulty step, it can sometimes be at least partly corrected by putting in a large amount of the facilitator. Homocysteinuria is one such disease. Since medical thinking looks at diseases as fairly discrete "entities," it was natural for doctors to figure that the vitamin treatment would work for the disease homocysteinuria but not for people with mild tendencies toward higher than normal levels of homocysteine.

Now, 30 years later, folic acid and vitamin B_6 treatment of mild elevations of homocysteine has been proven to be effective in preventing cardiovascular disease. Still, medical and public health authorities do not advocate the screening of individuals for higher than normal homocysteine levels and their treatment with vitamins because what has been "shown" had not been "proven." Only after the completion of a prospective blind trial of folic acid for the prevention of vascular disease will such a recommendation be made. Such an experiment is now under way in Oregon.[18] A senior member of the team carrying out the research is emphatic in stating that individuals should not rush to take folic acid supplements because they have not been proven safe and effective by the standards of a double-blind placebo controlled prospective study.[19]

The issues are very much the same as those associated with neural tube defects in which there was a 20-year lag between initial reliable reports of the relationship between folic acid needs and the risk of a woman bearing a child with a birth defect. Research proving the association between folic acid problems and neural tube defects was long and hard, and the same kind of proof, based on a prospective double-blind placebo controlled trial, is turning out to be even harder to carry out in the case of mild homocysteine elevations and the prevention of cardiovascular disease. It would be especially difficult from an ethical perspective.

Somehow the ethics of giving a placebo to pregnant women seemed acceptable to researchers even after it was clear that the placebo placed the recipients at a higher risk than those who got the folic acid. Those who make public health policy allowed women to be subjected to such an experiment in the name of good policy formation.

Now there is good evidence that those with high homocysteine levels would benefit from supplementation of folic acid, vitamin B_6 and, perhaps vitamin B_{12} for the prevention of cardiovascular disease. We should all be grateful to the many adults who are willing to take a placebo for years as part of an experiment that may show that they would get earlier-onset cardiovascular disease. Public health authorities are unlikely to recommend folic acid supplementation for individuals with mild elevations of homocysteine in the near future. In the meantime, it makes sense to select foods that are rich in folic acid and to take folic acid supplements as long as the supplementation poses no conceivable risk.

WHEN NOT TO TAKE FOLIC ACID SUPPLEMENTS

Mysterious misadventure with folic acid. Gladys Love is a 60-year-old woman whose dad died about eight years before she consulted me for depression. After her dad's death she became depressed in an unusual way. She cried all the time. Whenever she was alone or unobserved, the smallest stimulus would produce floods of tears that she blocked in public by sheer and exhausting willpower. To most of her friends, she was a vivacious and energetic person, and only a few intimate friends knew of her sadness. Her family life was stable and supportive, despite financial reverses that left her worried, but in no way poor. When she first described her plight to me, she hid her pain so well that I saw no clues that might indicate a biochemical basis for her sadness. In addition, she clearly acknowledged missing her father, who had been the mainstay of her life before his death.

I was guarded in suggesting that measuring certain aspects of her biochemical function might reveal a correctable problem, but based on many successful outcomes I have an optimism about this basic approach. I measured her levels of certain trace minerals and found a deficit of manganese. I also measured her urine amino acids as excreted over a 24-hour period and found a marked abnormality of certain amino acids that have to do with ridding the body of toxins (cysteine, cystine, cystathionine and methionine). I suggested supplements to correct the problems that were, in fact, uncovered. Within a week of beginning treatment, her problem cleared completely and the emotional makeup she had had before her illness was restored.

We went on to discuss various ideas I had to offer about

preventive nutrition, and I suggested, among other things, that she take 5 mg of folic acid daily. Within a few days of starting the folic acid her depression returned in a form that was identical to the one she had described to me at the time of our initial visit. It seemed to her that the folic acid supplement had precipitated the return of her tears. She discontinued the folic acid and her mood returned to normal. She restarted folic acid and reproduced the crash. She stopped again and returned again to normal. I am now in the process of trying to spot the biochemical quirk that makes her so susceptible to negative effects from folic acid, but given the limitations of tests for individual biochemical quirks, the odds are against solving the mystery.

Serious misadventure with folic acid. So, the first, and obvious, rule concerning intolerance to folic acid is that if it does not feel right, stop it. You can take comfort from the lack of any evidence that substantial amounts of folic acid can do harm without your knowing it with one important exception. There is a widespread medical opinion that large doses of folic acid may dangerously mask a deficiency of vitamin B_{12}. Formal documentation in the medical literature of actual cases of problems arising from the ingestion of folic acid by B_{12}-deficient individuals is shadowy. Dr. Butterworth polled more than 1200 specialists in order to find out the prevalence of neurological symptoms provoked in patients who have taken folic acid and created an imbalance in their B_{12} chemistry.[20] The survey, though scientifically informal, provided reassurance that the risk of creating B_{12} problems with folic acid is very low. Three probable cases were turned up in a sample that represented 10 years of clinical experience among 860 respondents to Dr. Butterworth's query.

But the stakes are high: permanent damage to nerves has been observed in people taking folic acid while neglecting to repair a serious deficiency of vitamin B_{12}. Therefore, to maximize safety one must be assured of a normal B_{12} status before consuming doses of folic acid in excess of 0.8 mg daily. A normal serum B_{12} level, available from any medical laboratory, provides a reasonable degree of certainty that one's B_{12} status is adequate. However, there is ample evidence that some individuals who have normal B_{12} blood levels may still benefit from B_{12} supplementation and may therefore be considered to have been functionally deficient. In such people the most sensitive indicator of vitamin B_{12} function, a plasma or serum level of methylmalonic acid, is required for documentation of the B_{12} abnormality. To be completely on the safe side before embarking on long-term folic acid supplementation at doses above 0.8 mg, I recommend that my patients have their methylmalonic acid levels checked.

Low dose alert. Some of us may be able to anticipate a negative reaction to taking even modest supplements of folic acid, say, 0.4 or 0.8 mg per day. Such persons were first described by Carl Pfeiffer, M.D., Ph.D., one of the pioneers in describing correlations between biochemical balance and mood and behavior. He was one of several psychiatrists who began to delve into the biochemistry of schizophrenia in the 1940s following the observation in the 1930s that psychotic states very similar to schizophrenia were caused by vitamin B_3 deficiency (pellagra). The pellagra model and the psychedelic effects of mescaline and LSD (discovered in 1937) made it clear that serious disorders of mood and perception were probably related to biochemical abnormalities and were not "emotional disorders" in the sense of being caused by early life experiences or faulty nurturing as many psychiatrists believed at the time.

Dr. Pfeiffer (who died in 1988) eventually founded the Princeton BioCenter in New Jersey where I worked in 1991 and 1992. Now a clinic serving the needs of patients with a variety of problems, the BioCenter was for years a center for the treatment of people suffering from various forms of schizophrenia.

Dr. Pfeiffer described variations of biochemical patterns in schizophrenics from whom he learned to identify in normal people a tendency called *histadelia*. Histadelia, which means high histamine, is a somewhat loose package of symptoms and traits that produce various levels of discomfort in different individuals: depression; allergies to pollen, mold, dust and other inhalants; compulsive behavior sometimes associated with workaholic habits; big hands and feet with long fingers and toes; a tendency to sweat, cry and produce mucous liberally. Such traits occur in various combinations and degrees in different individuals who also tend to be early risers and "fast metabolizers," which means they tolerate higher doses of medications, alcohol and recreational drugs more easily than the average person. One may have high histamine levels without suffering from any kind of disability. In fact, many high achievers have the profile of a high histamine chemistry. When the profile is accompanied by serious disorders of mood and perception, treatment with a combination of nutrients may be helpful. However, folic acid sometimes has negative effects in these individuals, exacerbating some symptoms such as depression.

When I asked Dr. Bonnie Camo, a former protégé of Dr. Pfeiffer and staff physician at the BioCenter, how frequently the folic acid problem actually arises in her patients, she said, "Not as often as Dr. Pfeiffer's writings and teachings have implied." Nonetheless, she feels that Dr. Pfeiffer's description of persons who may have a negative reaction to folic acid remains useful and that the problem may arise occasionally. She recommends multivitamins without folic acid for high histamine patients, but feels that people with a high histamine profile could experiment with folic acid as long as they are aware that it might increase any tendency to depression or allergies.

Drug interactions. Let us review the possible interactions of folic acid with certain medications. Folic acid works at such a fundamental level in the life activities of all living things that interfering with its function can be useful when we wish to interfere with the actions of a bacterium, a parasite or a cancer cell. When the bacterium, parasite or cancer cell is inside us, we have to figure out a way of harming the pest without poisoning ourselves when we take a drug that interferes with folic acid's functions. Folic acid antagonism is the mechanism of action in some medications you may have taken—for example, *trimethoprim* (an ingredient in Bactrim and Septra in which it is combined with a sulfa drug to form an antibacterial drug). It is less likely that you have taken *pyrimethamine,* a medication generally used to prevent or treat malaria, which is caused by a parasite. In both the antibacterial and antiparasitic drugs, the folic acid antagonism is achieved in the germ without injury to the person because the folic acid chemistry of the germ is sufficiently different that the drug can kill the germ without affecting human folic acid. Moreover, you can take folic acid supplements when taking these antimicrobial drugs without significantly interfering with the drug.

Antagonizing antagonists? Folic acid antagonists are also used to treat diseases in which a germ is not the direct cause—namely, cancer, leukemia, psoriasis, rheumatoid arthritis, polymyositis, dermatomyositis, Reiter's syndrome, Wegener's granulomatosis, sarcoidosis, primary biliary cirrhosis, hypertension, Crohn's disease, ulcerative colitis, gout and epilepsy. The drug methotrexate is given to some patients with cancers or certain leukemias. Sulfasalazine is used to treat Crohn's disease and ulcerative colitis. Triampterene is a blood pressure-lowering medication with some folic acid antagonism. There is no evidence to suggest that taking supplements of folic acid with any of these medications is harmful, in fact, Butterworth points out that there is some evidence that folic acid might combine beneficially with such medications.[22] It has now been accepted by experts in rheumatoid arthritis that combining folic acid with methotrexate treatment offers protection against some of the toxicity of the treatment without interfering with the symptom relief given by the methotrexate.[23]

Epilepsy treatment with phenytoin (Dilantin) presents a more complex question. On the one hand, phenytoin's capacity to inhibit folic acid has little or nothing to do with its ability to inhibit seizures. Individuals taking phenytoin should be monitored for folic acid deficiency and take supplements in sufficient quantities to avoid becoming deficient. There is some evidence to suggest that high doses of folic acid may increase brainwave abnormalities in individuals with seizure disorders. Doses of more than 0.8 mg per day of folic acid should be used only with medical supervision in individuals with seizure disorders whether or not they are taking phenytoin.

Colchicine, a medication that relieves the symptoms of gout, is a folic acid antagonist. Part of the way that it works may have to do with its suppression of folic acid metabolism in the patient. On the other hand, it may be that like sulfasalazine, folic acid should accompany colchicine in order to protect the patient from the negative effects of interfering with folic acid function.

Summary. There is more concern associated with the taking of drugs that may increase folic acid needs than with the possible harmful combination of folic acid with a particular drug. Long-term use of colchicine with folic acid has uncertain status. High-dose folic acid in combination with phenytoin may decrease thresholds for seizure activity. The benefit of taking folic acid with methotrexate for arthritis treatment has been established. The same may turn out to be true regarding the combination of folic acid and methotrexate for cancer treatment, but there is widespread medical opinion that folic acid should not be combined with methotrexate, and I would not advise you to do so without the approval of your doctor.

DISORDERS OF MOOD

In describing Dr. Pfeiffer's work, I referred to the beginnings of interest in the biochemistry of mood and behavior in the late 1930s. By the mid-1950s, Abraham Hoffer, Humphry Osmund, Carl Pfeiffer, John Smithies and others had begun to explore ways of diagnosing and treating patients with vitamin and mineral supplements to correct biochemical quirks. The focus was on treating the individual as opposed to treating the disease, which already placed their approach at odds with evolving trends in conventional psychiatry. Then, as now, a strong overriding impulse in conventional psychiatry was to refine processes for making a diagnosis with the logical assumption that better diagnosis would lead to better treatment as well as better communication among researchers who needed to agree on definitions. We can hardly carry out an intelligent conversation about people with various problems without having labels put on the problems, such as anxiety, depression, psychosis, mania, and hyperactivity. I cringe, however, when patients are told that the reason for their mood or behavior is that it is being *caused* by anxiety, depression and the like. Depression is the *name* of the problem and not the cause. Similarly, hyperactivity is a description of a child's behavior. It strikes me as odd that parents are asked to accept the explanation that their child's problem is being *caused* by hyperactivity.

Naming and blaming. Confusion between the name and the cause of a problem is more than a semantic issue. The confusion leads to very practical problems when medications enter the picture. The idea that a drug will treat a certain condition is very appealing. In many instances the idea is accurate: Aspirin and other pain relievers "treat" pain; sleeping pills "treat" insomnia; and antidepressant medications frequently elevate mood. Antibiotics kill germs that cause infections and thereby treat the infection. An antibiotic is much closer to being a real treatment of the underlying problem than is aspirin, which alleviates the pain without removing the cause of the pain.

Most of the drugs used for the treatment of problems of mood, perception, behavior and attention are more like aspirin than antibiotics: They alleviate the symptom without correcting the cause. When drugs work very well to alleviate symptoms with little risk, their appeal is justified, but if a medication silences a message from one's body that an imbalance needs repair, then the medicine postpones or prevents more appropriate measures to correct the imbalance.

The possible effect of naturally occurring substances on the mood of certain individuals is more and more likely to be ignored as the taking of mood-altering drugs becomes more widespread. The current enthusiasm for using mood-altering medications is matched by the longstanding disdain of conventional psychiatry for nutritional treatments. The 1972 position paper of the American Psychiatric Association condemned "megavitamin therapy," and the position statement still serves as armor for psychiatrists who take the attitude that "all that stuff about vitamins has been discredited." In my opinion, the authors of the 1972 position statement did not do their homework in consulting the authorities and written materials available at the time. Since 1972, there has been an ongoing accumulation of scientific information describing a rich and complex interaction between diet, supplements, deficiencies and individual biochemical quirks on the one hand and problems in mood, behavior, perception and attention on the other. Part of the emerging picture has to do with vitamins to correct deficiencies, and another part has to do with vitamins used in higher doses to treat quirks in individual biochemistry.

The nervous system is a busy system. The folic acid needs of various tissues rise with the general level of activity of the tissues. Because the central nervous system is metabolically very active, it is not surprising that various studies have implicated folic acid abnormalities in mood and other disturbances of nervous system function. A recent review[24] of folic acid in psychiatric disorders tabulated the results of 14 studies of folic acid in psychiatric disorders published between 1967 and 1992. More than 2800 patients from the United Kingdom, France and the United States were included in reports which described the folic acid levels of patients admitted to psychiatric facilities. The incidence of folic acid deficiency varied from 18 percent of the patients studied to rates as high as 80 to 90 percent in the very elderly populations studied. The crux of the review is that folic acid deficiency is very common among patients being admitted to the hospital for psychiatric conditions, especially depression and dementia. Dependence on simple blood counts to identify the kind of anemia often associated with folic acid deficiency was not sufficient to detect patients with significant deficiency. Measures of red blood cell folic acid were the most reliable.

The full implications of the correlations found between low folic acid levels and higher degrees of mental impairment remain to be explored. It is possible, for example, that those with lower levels of folic acid became deficient because their impairment interfered with proper diet. On the other hand, there was clear evidence that improvement of mental impairment occurred with folic acid supplementation. Treatment with folic acid often required months to reach its full effect. In another review[25] of the subject, Iris Bell, M.D., Ph.D., Professor of Psychiatry at the University of Arizona, maintains that the patients with the lowest folic acid levels had the poorest tests for cognitive function and that supplementation gave rise to improvements in memory test scores. She also points out that both the clinical and laboratory evidence for folic acid deficiency may be subtle and require special tests such as those for serum homocysteine.

In another more general review[26] of nutritional factors associated with aging and the loss of cognitive function, Irwin H. Rosenberg of the U.S. Department of Agricultural Human Nutrition Research Center on Aging at Tufts University in Boston makes a strong plea for using homocysteine levels to screen for folic acid (and B_6 and B_{12}) problems in the elderly. He uses much the same approach as I have already described—that is, using homocysteine levels as a way of looking for people at risk for cardiovascular disease. Again, the question is "How old, depressed or demented do I need to become before wanting to measure my homocysteine levels?" Again, the answer may depend on whether one views it from the private or public policy perspective.

Histapenia and folic acid. I have already referred to the possibility that some individuals with high histamine levels might not do well with folic acid supplements. What about people with low histamine levels, which is what is meant by the term *histapenia*? Such individuals have a profile that is opposite to that of the high histamine person. Folic acid is part of a complex strategy for helping unwell low histamine persons improve their chemical balance and reduce or eliminate symptoms. The complexity of the strategy[27] is a good reminder that the use of nutritional supplements usually involves more than one at a time. Folic acid's functions are closely tied with vitamin B_{12} and vitamin B_6. Vitamin B_6's functions are closely tied with magnesium. Magnesium and vitamin B_6 have a role in nearly every aspect of biochemistry, which itself is an enormous web of interacting systems.

An elderly person who is depressed or confused may benefit from evaluation of his or her folic acid status. However, folic acid deficiency usually does not appear in isolation from other deficiencies.

FOOD SOURCES OF FOLIC ACID

Some otherwise healthy foods are poor sources of folic acid while others have surprising concentrations. A study of the following table taken from a nutritional computer database will speak for itself.

Unfortunately, cooking foods may remove as much as 90 percent of the folic acid. Moreover, the bioavailability of folic acid from various foods may vary from 60 percent in cow's milk to 30 percent in orange juice, depending on how different forms of folic acid are handled in the digestive tract. Grains are not a particularly rich source of folic acid, so breakfast cereals achieve a high folic acid rating through fortification. It should also be noted that alcohol is an antagonist of folic acid, and alcohol abuse is one of the main causes of severe folic acid deficiency.

Best Dietary Sources of Folic Acid*

Amount	*Food*	*mcg of Folic Acid*
1 oz	Brewer's yeast	1109
1 cup	*Total* breakfast cereal	400
3 oz	Beef liver, cooked	187
3 oz	Raw spinach	166
1	Avocado (Florida)	162

3 oz	Cooked spinach	124
3 oz	Cooked frozen sliced okra	124
3 oz	Endive	121
1	Avocado (California)	113
3 oz	Kidney beans, cooked	110
3 oz	Turnip greens, cooked	101
3 oz	Raw bok choy cabbage	84
3 oz	Asparagus spears, cooked	83
3 oz	Beef kidney, cooked	83
3 oz	Beets, cooked	73
1	Artichoke, cooked	62
3 oz	Peas, cooked	57
1 oz	Watercress	57
3 oz	Walnuts	57
3 oz	Cauliflower, cooked	56
1 oz	Wakame seaweed	54
3 oz	Brussels sprouts, cooked	52
3 oz	Parsnips, cooked	50
3 oz	Almonds	50

*Food Processor II ESHA Research.

MEASURING FOLIC ACID

One way to find out whether a nutrient can improve your health is to take some of it and see what happens. Such an approach has some merit when applied to certain kinds of nutritional supplementation, but it does not have much of a place as concerns folic acid. The best reason against it is that fatigue is the main symptom you might wish to monitor during your experimental taking of folic acid. Fatigue could be the result of many problems, including a vitamin B_{12} deficiency, which would be a very good reason not to take folic acid without first taking B_{12}, for the reasons discussed earlier.

Another way to find out about your excess folic acid needs is to keep track of everything you eat and look up its folic acid content in a nutrition reference book or a computer program that helps you calculate the nutritional content of your food. Blood tests measure folic acid in two different parts of the blood: in the serum or within the red blood cells. The serum is an indicator of short-term folic acid deficiency, within the recent week or so. Red blood cells, which have a life span of about four months, are "born" with a certain content of folic acid when they are first made in the bone marrow. Their folic acid content represents a more stable pool of folic acid in the body and is an indicator of longer term folic acid deficiency. It is the preferred measure.

Urine and/or serum homocysteine levels indicate whether a certain crucial function of folic acid is being carried out. High levels of homocysteine show that you have a special need for folic acid and/or vitamin B_6. The special need may not be reflected in low-serum or red blood cell folic acid levels. High levels of homocysteine are a marker for a high risk for cardiovascular and other illnesses. I think most people should have their homocysteine levels checked at some point as a way of assessing their risk. The most sensitive way of assessing homocysteine is following the ingestion of the amino acid methionine. The test, called a methionine-loaded homocysteine level, is conducted by taking 20 mg of methionine per kg of body weight in four divided doses during the collection of a 24-hour urine specimen.

FOLIC ACID IN ITS PLACE

Now that you understand why folic acid is such an important nutrient and why many people would benefit from eating foods rich in folic acid and taking folic acid supplements, please remember that folic acid is not the answer to everything. Of the six major activities in biochemistry, folic acid figures heavily in three: single-carbon transfers, waste disposal and messenger molecules. Other nutrients have key roles in the other functions. For example, vitamins B_1, B_2, B_6, pantothenic acid, magnesium and others play important roles in the disassembly of fuel molecules to produce energy. Vitamins C, E, beta carotene, selenium, vitamin B_3, vitamin B_2 and others are nutrients indispensable for antioxidant function. Essential fatty acids and various vitamins and minerals are critical to the formation and maintenance of flexible cell membranes and to the synthesis of prostanoid hormones.

Whatever we know about chemistry and all of the important roles of folic acid, the overriding importance of individuality is what I confront every day as a physician. Folic acid is life-saving to some of us, preventive of certain kinds of mischief in others and may not agree with a few. If you were in my office and I could examine you and do certain kinds of tests on your blood or urine, I would have a better, though still imperfect, understanding of how your individual biochemistry might influence your choice of foods and supplements to improve or sustain your health. As it is, in writing this booklet I have to refer to factors in biochemistry that are reliably the same from person to person. All of us are dependent on certain substances that account for the "goodness" in foods, that is, the essential minerals, vitamins, amino acids and fatty acids.

When I began my training as a physician, I learned that the essential nutrients had critical roles in biochemistry, but the message that came with that learning, and in my subsequent training, was that nutrients are trivial compared with drugs. "Real" doctors prescribe drugs. Nutrients were considered wimpy by comparison. Such attitudes still prevail in mainstream medical practice, despite a rich body of scientifically validated evidence supporting the curative and protective effects of various nutrients.

As of this writing, no nutrient can compete with folic acid for the premier place among substances that are safe, inexpensive and powerful in helping many individuals gain and sustain health.

REFERENCES

1. Rosenberg, I. H. and Mason, J. B. Folate, dysplasia, and cancer [editorial]. *Gastroenterology* 1989, Aug; 97 (2):502–503.
2. Whitehead, N., Reyner, F. and Lindenbaum, J. Megaloblastic changes in the cervical epithelium: association with oral contraceptive therapy and reversal with folic acid. *JAMA* 1973; 226:1421–1424.
3. Butterworth, C. E., Jr., Hatch, K. D., Gore, H., Mueller, H. and Krumdieck, C. L. Improvement in cervical dysplasia associated with folic acid therapy in users of oral contraceptives. *Am J Clin Nutr.* 1982; 35: 73–82.
4. Butterworth, C. E., Jr., Hatch, K. D., Soong, S., Cole, P., Tamura, T., Sauberlich, H., Borst, M., Macaluso, M. and Baker, V. Oral folic acid supplementation for cervical dysplasia: a clinical intervention trial. *Am J Obstet Gynecol.* 1992; 166:803–809.
5. Butterworth, C. E., Jr., Hatch, K. D., Macaluso, M., Cole, P., Sauberlich, H. E., Soong, S., Borst, M. and Baker, V. Folate deficiency and cervical dysplasia. *JAMA* 1992; 267:931–934.
6. Ibid.
7. Butterworth, C. E., Jr. Interactions of nutrients with oral contraceptives and other drugs. *J Am Diet Assoc.* 1973; 62:51–54.
8. Lashner, B. A., Heidenreich, P. A., Su, G. L., Kane, S. V. and Hanauer, S. B. Effect of folate supplementation on the incidence of dysplasia and cancer in chronic ulcerative colitis. A case-control study. *Gastroenterology* 1989, Aug; 97(2):255–259.
9. Jaskiewicz, K., Marasas, W. F. O., Lazarus, C., Beyers, A. D. and Van Helden, P. D. Association of esophageal cytological abnormalities with vitamin and lipotrope deficiencies in populations at risk for esophageal cancer. *Anticancer Res.* 1988; 1:711–716.

10. Heimberger, D. Localized deficiencies of folic acid in areo-digestive tissues. *Ann NY Acad Sci.* 1992; 669:87–95.
11. Smithells, R. W., Sheppard, S. and Schorah, C. J. Vitamin deficiencies and neural tube defects. *Arch Dis Child* 1976, Dec; 51(12):944–950.
12. MRC Vitamin Study Research Group. Prevention of neural tube defects: results of the Medical Research Council Vitamin Study. *Lancet* 1991, Jul; 338 (8760):131–137.
13. Czeizel, A. E. and Dudas, I. Prevention of the first occurrence of neural-tube defects by periconceptional vitamin supplementation. *N Engl J Med* 1992, Dec 4; 327(26):1832–1835.
14. Brattstrom, I., Israelsson, B., Norrving, B., Bergqvist, D., Thorne, J., Hultberg, B. and Hamfelt, A. Impaired homocysteine metabolism in early-onset cerebral and peripheral occlusive arterial disease. Effects of pyridoxine and folic acid treatment. *Atherosclerosis* 1990, Feb; 81(1):51–60.
15. Ellis, J. M. and McCully, K. S. Decreased incidence of acute myocardial infarction from vitamin B_6 therapy. Submitted for publication.
16. Jacobsen, D. W., et al. Rapid HPLC determination of total homocysteine and other thiols in serum and plasma: sex difference and correlation with cobalmin and folate concentrations in healthy subjects. *Clin Chem.* 1994; 40:873–881.
17. Butterworth, C. E., Jr., Krumdieck, C. L. and Baugh, C. M. Studies on the absorption and metabolism of folic acid. II. Homocysteinuria. *Ala J Med Sci.* 1971; 8:1; 30–43.
18. Malinow, M. R., Kang, S. S., Taylor, L. M., Wong, P. W., Coull, B., Inahara, T., Mukerjee, D., Sexton, G. and Upson, B. Prevalence of hyperhomocyst(e)inemia in patients with peripheral arterial occlusive disease. *Circulation* 1989, Jun; 79(6):1180–1188.
19. Taylor, L. M., Jr. Presentation given at American College for Advancement in Medicine, San Diego, November 1994.
20. Butterworth, C. E., Jr. and Tamura, T. Folic acid safety and toxicity: a brief review. *Am J Clin Nutr.* 1989; 50:2; 353–358.
21. Ibid.
22. Ibid.
23. Stewart, K. A., et al. Folate supplementation in methotrexate-treated rheumatoid arthritis patients. Seminars in Arthritis and Rheumatism. April 1991; 20(5):332–338. Morgan, S., et al. Folate

supplementation and methotrexate. *Annals of Rheumatic Diseases* 1993; 52:315–316.

24. Crellin, R., Bottiglieri, T. and Reynolds, E. H. Folate and psychiatric disorders: clinical potential. *Drugs,* 1993; 45(5):623–636.
25. Bell, I. R. Vitamin B_{12} and folate in acute geropsychiatric patients. *The Nutrition Report* 1991, Jan; 9(1):1, 8.
26. Rosenberg, I. H. and Miller, J. W. Nutritional factors and physical and cognitive functions of elderly people. *Am J Clin Nutr.* 1992; 55:1237–43S.
27. Jaffe, R. and Kruesi, O. The biological-immunology window: a molecular view of psychiatric management. *International Clinical Nutrition Review* 1992, Jan; 12(1):9–26.
28. Heber, D., et al. Biennial survey of physician clinical-nutrition training programs. *Am J Clin Nutr.* 1993; 57:463–469.